THE ONE DAY DIET

How to Live a Cancer Prevention Lifestyle

EVAN MONEY

www.theonedaydiet.com

ISBN: 1449916783
ISBN-13: 9781449916787

"Evan Money is one of those rare individuals who puts his beliefs into action; he will teach you to do the same. Evan walks the walk and that is what makes him so special. He has my highest recommendation!"

Dr. Keith Phillips - President, World Impact

"Evan's personality contagiously inspires everyone who comes in contact with him. His focused and dedicated approach motivates and encourages others to maximize their own individual abilities and realize positive growth in their lives, and leads them to be the best at what they do."

Jeff Harlow - Arena Football Team Owner / Boxing Promoter

"I have known Evan and his family for years. Honest, Creative, Dynamic, Expressive, when Evan speaks you want to listen. He thinks big, dreams big and then he moves and makes his dreams a reality. Adding action to ideas? - Evan lives it. If you can catch just a little of his fire, a little of his passion, it could make life oh so much more interesting."

Dr. Douglas Holtzinger - *Founder, Back Care Institute*

To contact Evan for speaking engagements call:
1-877-WOW-EVAN
or e-mail:
evan@evanmoney.com
www.evanmoney.com

First off, I need to give a big Thank You to God for being so patient with me. I'm very thankful He allows U-turns in life.

Secondly, I need to thank my bride, Susan Money, for giving up her role as a strong woman and choosing to become a woman of strength.

Lastly, thank you to everyone who has ever encouraged me in my life; a kind word can go a long way.

———— ❧ ————

"Experts and Educators thrive on making simple things complicated, Communicators make complicated things simple."
– Dr. John C. Maxwell

CHAPTER 1

The great news about this book is that it's for real and it's easier than you think. The most important point I want to make right upfront is that <u>this is so simple</u>. Life is too hectic to worry about counting calories, counting carbs, weighing your chicken, or all that other diet fad nonsense. All great things are simple; the "One Day Diet" is about simplicity and about getting you results. The best part is you will be automatically preventing cancer, with no extra effort. If you find this hard to believe simply read on and discover the truth.

In my first book "Take Action Now- How to Live Your Dream in 3 Weeks", I hinted at this book in Chapter 9. In it, I talked about how too many people get intimidated with starting something new or simply just changing. The secret, of course, is just working on today. Take Michael Phelps for example, the guy who won a historic 8 gold medals in the 2008 summer Olympics. Most people think he trained for 4 years, and that is simply not true. He only trained for one day! Let me explain. He made a decision every day. When he woke up every morning, he had a simple choice to make: train or don't train. He simply chose each day to show up at the pool. He could not train a day in advance; he could not say, "Oh, I think I'll train for Tuesday and Wednesday since I'm already here." Michael Phelps, Tiger Woods, Michael Jordon or any greatest-of-all-time-athletes have this in common with you: they can only train today.

It's the same with your current diet. You can simply choose today to eat an apple or a doughnut. That's it; it's a one day diet plan. See how simple this is; just make a decision that today you will make better food choices. Remember the saying: "An apple a day keeps the doctor away." Right? What if it's true? As the legendary Jim Rohn would say, "If you confuse the apple a day with the doughnut a day, it's a recipe for disaster."

John Maxwell says, **"You will never change your life until you change something daily."** This statement is so true; everyone thinks change is some big process, like quitting smoking. You don't need to quit smoking forever. In fact you can't; you can only not smoke today. It is the same with alcohol, internet porn or any addiction. You can never quit drinking or quit porn forever; just choose not to do it today. See how the pressure comes off you? You just tell yourself, "I'm not quitting smoking, because nobody likes a quitter anyway." (LOL!) You are just making a choice to not smoke today.

So with this "today" theme, I'm going to show how simple the "One Day Diet" is and how fast you will get results. In this book we will cover 5 simple Keys that make the "One Day Diet" work. What great tasting things you can eat, when to eat them, genetics and how they work for you, why you don't need exercise to lose weight and a few other surprises like preventing cancer.

Before we get into the details, let me share a little bit about my journey in the health and fitness world and how I have been able to put this all together for you.

I grew up in the pre-video game era; well, you could call Atari and Colecovision video games I guess, but compared to what is out there today, they hardly qualify. So needless to say, I was an active boy who rode his bike everywhere, played sports, surfed and skateboarded. Child obesity was an unknown back then; it just didn't happen because for the most part kids were physically active.

As I grew up, I dreamed of playing professional football, however when I got into high school, it became apparent that everyone had already started growing except me. In fact, when I graduated at 17 I was 150 pounds soaking wet and about 5'8". Not exactly what Division I football coaches were looking for, or any football coach for that matter! Finally, when I was about 19, I reached my full height of 5'11" and I was lean and a muscular 170 pounds. At the age of 21, a buddy invited me to a gym to workout and I got "hooked." From that day on I was in the gym training 5 to 6 days a week for approximately the next 10 years.

My results were incredible. In about 5 years I was 200 pounds of solid muscle on my 5'11" frame.

I was accused many times of being on steroids; actually, it was a great compliment to me since protein shakes were about the only supplement I used. For those 10 years, I read and tested every type of diet and exercise regimen, all in the hopes of being a professional bodybuilder. I thought if I just worked hard enough I could get my body to do what it was genetically incapable of doing.

I finally woke up to reality after I started getting a barrage of injuries; all I really accomplished in those 10 years was severely overtraining my body. Today I'm still paying the price. The old saying that "Football is a young man's game," really applies here because football, just like too much weightlifting, is very damaging to your body. You just don't know how damaging until years later. However, this whole process is what led me to dedicate 18 years researching diet and exercise alternatives as well as optimum health and cancer prevention. Over this time I have been able to test and experiment on myself and family to perfect what I'm going to teach you.

Unlike overweight celebrity talk show hosts or diet experts that do not practice what they preach,

I have personally tested and live out everything I'm teaching you about. So you don't have to make all the mistakes I have; you just get the distilled information on what I have discovered to be the best for a lean, healthy and cancer free body.

Lastly, and this truth is huge, I want you to understand that the "One Day Diet" is a process. Some of you are an all-or-nothing type; you want to do it all and get the maximum results in the minimum amount of time. Others may just want to ease into this; the great news is you can do it any way you want. It's totally up to you; the best part is you will get results no matter what.

The most common mistakes I see people make are the "crash diet" or the present fad diets, where they totally change everything and do get results, but 3 months later, they are back to their old habits and they regain all the weight. Now part of this has nothing to do with food and part of it does, so we are going to cover both sides of the coin and get you permanent results. Are you ready to take action and get started? Ok, here we go!

ACTION STEPS:

#1 Find a picture in a magazine of what you want your body to look like. Cut it out and post it somewhere you will see it every day.

#2 Start with the apple a day theory, just decide you will eat one apple sometime today. You may want to go to the store and buy 7 or 8 apples so you can have them available.

---

*"I didn't know I had a headache
until the pain stopped."*

CHAPTER 2

WHAT TO EAT & WHEN

Gary Player, one of golf's all time greatest legends, was playing in his final Masters Tournament in 2009. Gary is 73 years old and is known the world over for his overall health and stamina. How many 73-year-olds do you know that can play 18 rounds of golf without using a cart? As he was signing autographs, Gary was overheard explaining the keys to his longevity, and he said the following, "No bacon, no milk, no white bread and very little ice cream."

Pretty simple isn't it. There is a little more to it, but most health and nutrition books all agree that there are certain foods that simply are not worth eating. What's amazing about the "One Day Diet" is that you can continue to eat whatever you want and still get results. Let me explain:

The first key to the "One Day Diet" is what to eat and when, if you only do this one key you will boost your health and fitness levels 1,000% over the average American. If you follow the other keys you will be on your way to giving Gary Player and even Jack Lalanne a run for their money on terms of health.

SO HERE IS KEY #1:
Only eat fruit from the time you wake up until 12 noon!

Eat as much as you want, whenever you want. Smoothies are fine, frozen blueberries and bananas are my favorites; you can add water or ice. The great thing about fruit is you can grab it and go; it's the ultimate fast food. Bananas are the best for me because they hold me over longer than say watermelon. However, it does not matter. Eat as much as you like whenever you like. EAT ONLY FRUIT UNTIL NOON.

Of course you should still drink water!!! And lots of it! If you have not figured out…the key to ageless skin and hair is to be hydrated. Ask Tina Turner, the legendary singer, her beauty secret and she will tell you she drinks a lot of water. You want to drop 20 years off your appearance? Add 2 quarts of water a day(that's only 4 tall glasses) and watch what happens.

Please note: DO NOT DRINK FRUIT JUICE, unless you make it yourself, fresh squeezed. All bottled juice is heat pasteurized which kills all the live enzymes and just makes it empty calories. You still need to eat most of your fruit, so if you are going to fresh squeeze, then I recommend no more than 25% of your fruit to be juiced and the other 75% to be eaten.

Do this for 2 weeks solid and watch how much "crap" (literally) your body flushes from your system; some of you it may take 3 weeks because of all the garbage you have in your body. This will detoxify your body big time, so be ready for the "detox blues." You may feel slightly ill for a few days; not sick enough to stay home, but just not 100% normal. Also you will be spending some quality time in the bathroom as your body will literally be removing toxins it has been holding onto for a long time.

Let me repeat myself, so you are clear: Eat as much fruit as you want as often as you want from the time you wake up until12 noon. Apple pie does not count as fruit! DO NOT STARVE YOURSELF! Eat. Eat and Eat. Think of fruit as free food. It does not count against you. If you are hungry 10 or 20 minutes later, eat some more fruit. It's OK; this is the time to "splurge" as they say. As long as you're only eating uncooked, fresh raw fruit, (not from a can,) you are fine. (It is OK if you peel the skins off.) The first few days you will be surprised at how much fruit you are eating; you will be thinking it's not possible to eat this much and still lose weight. Trust me; you will be dropping weight like a ship drops an anchor, but you have to eat whenever you get hungry. After a few days or perhaps a week your body will start to adjust and you will not be eating as much, so don't worry.

Here is my daily routine to give you an idea of how this works. I wake up about 8am or 9am. I do not own an alarm clock, I simply wake up when I'm done sleeping. (I highly recommend this and "yes" I do have children). I usually eat a kiwi, an apple and 2 bananas when I first wake up. An hour or two later, I have a smoothie with frozen blueberries, (or raspberries, blackberries, cherries, or a berry mix) and 2 more bananas. At 12 noon I have a snack of oatmeal or a raw food bar, and I eat a regular lunch around 1 or 2pm, then a snack at 3 or 4pm of some raw nuts or popcorn or graham crackers, then a full dinner (a raw green salad, a protein, and some carbohydrates) at 5:30 or 6pm; I may have another snack of fruit before bed, if I stay up past 11pm.

For those that are wondering: "Yes, I eat like this every day, rain or shine, on the road or at home." If you are someone like my beautiful Bride, who loves diversity, you can have different fruits every day; bananas, kiwis and apples are just my favorites, so they are what I choose most often. You can get as exotic as you want with fruits from around the world, or you can just stick to the basics. The only rule is: <u>Eat fruit only from the time you wake up until 12 noon. Eat as much as you want, whenever you want.</u>

For some of you that are still skeptical, let me help you understand the benefits of raw fruit. What makes fruit so amazing is that it has its own live enzymes which help your body to digest it instead of using up your own enzymes, so you could look at fruit as being pre-digested food. (This is the reason you typically get hungry shortly after eating fruit.) Your body is able to absorb it and process it quickly. The vitamins in fruit are absorbed instantly and your body does not have to work to break them down.

Another great benefit is that fruits are packed with antioxidants; don't worry I won't launch into a sermon of how beneficial antioxidants are. I will however share this fun story with you about the day I was tested for my antioxidant level. I was walking into my gym and the head sales guy asked how my antioxidants were doing. I replied "Joe, I live an antioxidant lifestyle," his response was a laugh and he asked if I wanted to be tested. I agreed. I was hooked up to a laptop with some wimpy gauge on my finger. The gals giving me the test were nice enough and I soon figured out they were selling supplements. They were giving this FREE test, of course, to demonstrate and prove to the potential client how low their antioxidant levels were so they would buy their supplements. After the tested ended and my score came up, the first girl said, "Oh my God!" and the second girl ran over to see why she was so shocked. They told me I had the highest score they had ever seen. They were a little happy for me, but mostly sad because I wasn't going to buy any of their vitamins that day. It was actually very amusing to me that they just validated my healthful diet, even though they were trying to prove the contrary. This was just another added benefit of eating fruit everyday!

If you're looking for more details on how and why fruits are so beneficial, there are a million blogs, health journals and magazines to give you all the details you need.

Your next question may be: Why do I have to do this in the morning? Good question. In fact, there are people called "fruitarians," all they eat is fruit. These people may be the definition of too much of a good thing, but only time will tell. For the "One Day Diet" the reason we say only eat fruit until noon is because of the natural cycles of your body. If you don't "believe" in cycles then you have not spent any time with the female race. Every 28 days they have a cycle and in some cases it can be pretty intense. The tides, the solar system, the seasons all have cycles and your body works the same way.

CYCLE #1: ELIMINATION CYCLE OR "DETOX" (4am - 12 noon)

This is the time that your body naturally eliminates and detoxifies itself. Most of you reading this have no clue of this because your body is so filled with toxins from the crap food you're eating, in addition to your stress level and your lack of exercise. So trust me, your body is attempting to detoxify itself, but after you stack so much unhealthy food in your body, it has a hard time keeping up. The old adage of "I didn't know I had a headache until the pain stopped" fits here perfectly. Once you start on this program you soon find the cycles of your body and work with them.

CYCLE #2: EATING & DIGESTION
(12 noon - 8pm)

This is the best time for you to eat "real food" as some would say. This is when your body is at its peak to consume and digest heavier foods like grains, vegetables and meats. The goal here is not to run to McDonalds at noon and order a Big Mac every day. The goal is to eat 3 or 4 small to medium sized meals from 12 noon until 8pm. If you are anything like me and you love food, you just need to realize it's better to eat smaller meals more often than only one or two big meals. Your body just functions better that way, trust me. There have been numerous health studies that prove a reduced calorie diet adds longevity to life. There are other theories that explain this by simply saying your body has a set number of digestive enzymes and when you run out, you die. It really doesn't matter; the fact is that your body works and runs at its best when you eat smaller meals more frequently.

CYCLE #3: ABSORBTION (8pm - 4am)

This is when your body absorbs and assimilates the food you consumed during Cycle #2. The better food choices you make, the easier it is for your body to function, and the less waste you have. To give you an example: your body really is like a car. Most of us at one time or another have owned a crappy car that we didn't really take care of. After driving it for a while, you just get used to how bad it performs, until you drive a newer car or a car that has been well taken care of. Then the difference is night and day. You may relate better to driving on old worn out tires and then the day you get new tires you can really feel the difference. Then we always say, "If I knew it was that bad I would have gotten new tires sooner."

Our bodies are the same way; we can abuse them with smoking, drugs, alcohol, stress and no exercise and it still functions. However, our bodies break down so gradually we hardly notice how bad it is until we hit rock bottom. Just like with a car that has not been taken care of, one day the engine just blows, or in the case or our bodies, one day the whole thing just shuts down.

Don't let this happen to you. Take Action Now and make a quality decision to put better foods into your body.

(For more information about the digestion cycles of our bodies, see <u>Fit for Life</u> by Harvey and Marilyn Diamond.)

ACTION STEPS:

#1 Stock up on fruit today so you will have enough to follow through with eating fruit only until noon every day.

#2 Plan ahead on taking fruits with you that are not as messy as others for when you go to work, or wherever you travel before noon every day. Eat the messy ones at home.

"Eat to live, don't live to eat."
— Benjamin Franklin

CHAPTER 3

FOODS TO AVOID

A s we talked about in the first chapter, if all you did was just eat fruit until noon and then ate total crap food for the rest of the day, you would be 1,000 times better off than you are now. However, if you want the total prize and you want to look 10 or 20 years younger than you do, if you want to see your abs again or get into the best physical shape of your life, then it's time to use Key #2 of the "One Day Diet." This key is also simple: avoid the foods that are literally killing you. Keep in mind it's totally up to you how far you want to go with this, but if you go all the way, you will get the best results. It took me a long time to adapt my lifestyle to avoid all the foods I'm going to list below. Please understand for most of you it's a process, a daily choice. This is a marathon, not a sprint. Sure, there are a few hard core people who will immediately take action on everything I talk about, but you don't have to. The goal is to simply make progress. It may take you 6 months or 6 years but it doesn't matter. You choose the time frame; some of you may have some serious side effects from giving up these unhealthful foods. If that is the case, then make a gradual departure. You know your body better than anyone, so <u>listen to it</u>.

Make sure you understand the concept of withdrawal symptoms and cravings. You may have read or even experienced firsthand battling a drug or alcohol addiction. As you begin to break away and free your body of these toxins, what begins to happen is your body starts to crave the very thing that is destroying it. You will experience some of these very same feelings with certain foods. If that's the case, then I recommend a gradual decline. For example, if you choose to give up a certain food that you used to eat every day, start eating it only 5 days a week, then 3, then 2 etc…

SO HERE IS KEY #2:

Avoid the foods below!

FAST FOOD:
If it has a drive thru window, do not eat there.

I know the fast food places have started to see the light and they have lots of salads and grilled chicken, even Kentucky Fried Chicken has grilled chicken now! The challenge is the food is still so processed and heavily laden with salt, it really does not benefit your body at all to eat it. I'm not going to launch into a whole chapter here, so if you want more details on how bad fast food really is I recommend the book <u>Fast Food Nation</u> by Eric Schlosser. This book is a real eye-opener on the food processing industry, from meat-packing to food flavoring and additives. Or, to get another wakeup call on fast food, watch the movie "Super Size Me" (2004).

The surest way to really understand just how bad fast food is for you is to not eat it at all for 6 months, and then go have a full meal of it and you will literally spit it out; your senses will be so assaulted by the salt and preservatives it will amaze you. Even if you do eat it you will feel so lousy for the rest of the day and the next day, (because your body then tries to get rid of it), that you will never go back.

The best way to avoid fast food is to plan ahead. Pack a turkey sandwich on sprouted bread with mustard or a "RAW" almond butter and "RAW" honey sandwich (my favorite!) and some carrot or celery sticks.

It really is a simple process. Once you make the decision, your body will thank you.

RED MEAT!
__Eat Chicken, Turkey or Fish only.__

The health dangers of red meat and pork have been covered by so many researchers it's common knowledge that it contributes to high blood pressure, diabetes, heart challenges of all kinds, and obesity, to name only a few. Chicken, turkey and fish are much "cleaner" foods and easier for your body to digest and process. Does this mean you should never eat a steak or BBQ ribs again? No! However, you would be doing yourself a huge favor if you ate grass-feed and hormone-free beef. Yes, it's more expensive and harder to find, but your body will again thank you.

When talking about the "cost" of certain foods, a great comparison would be like driving a Ferrari and then putting cheap low octane gas in it. You know what will happen: the car will run poorly for a few days, or until all the cheap gas is used up. Will the car blow up instantly? No, of course not; it will just run at a much lower performance level. So, if you really want red meat that bad once in a while, then have it. Normally, when you remove an unhealthy food from your diet, your body then gets accustomed to not having to process it anymore, and if you go back and have that food again, let's just say, "Your stomach will let you know you made a poor choice." Ultimately, you will get to the point where it's just not worth it.

For example; my Bride was recently at a women's event at our church and they had all kinds of foods that she and I gave up years ago. However, she decided she wanted to indulge in the foods, and she happily savored all the tastes. The challenge was when she got home she did not feel well. In fact, the whole rest of the evening and the next day she felt like... I think the professional term is "crapola." She was amazed at how much it knocked her body out of rhythm. You see the cleaner you eat, the more you notice how negatively toxins affect you. So the next time my Bride is in that situation where she finds herself surrounded by foods we do not eat, she simply has to judge if these food choices are really worth the repercussions.

Dairy Products
COW'S MILK IS FOR COWS!

When this simple truth finally dawned on me I couldn't believe how ill-advised I was. For years I listened to the media on how wonderful dairy is and I ate it up, literally. However, after taking a break from dairy products, I noticed my digestion improved 500%. I no longer had a stuffy nose and I decreased the time that I spent on the toilet by

80%. My body literally transformed itself and I haven't looked back since.

For some of you, giving up dairy is like giving up life itself. I understand. My Bride was raised on cheese; her father was born in Europe and cheese was a way of life. She didn't totally give up cheese until a few years ago; it wasn't until she decided she wanted her amazing abs back. She cut down by about 80% and reaped the benefits. So when she ate it once or twice a week, she could really enjoy it. For her it was a choice between abs and cheese and she chose her abs. Now she is at the point of no return, 100% cheese-free and she is feeling and looking much better for it.

Incidentally, her father just recently gave up cheese, but sadly for him it wasn't until after he had a heart attack. He had to get his chest sawed open and have a quintuple bypass in order to come to the realization that dairy simply isn't worth the price we pay.

Again, I have nothing against the Dairy Council, or cows for that matter. In fact, one of my favorite foods is wood-fired BBQ chicken pizza, so believe me I understand. I just made the decision that BBQ chicken pizza just wasn't worth it anymore. The choice is up to you. Trust me, you are better off without dairy.

If you are still holding out and wondering about protein, calcium or other nutrients that dairy products provide, I understand. There are plenty of other food sources that provide these and are non-dairy, such as: beans, nuts, whole grains, and surprisingly, many vegetables like tomatoes, peppers, onions, sweet and dill pickles, broccoli, bok choy, celery, spinach, collard greens and kale, just to name a few. I also recommend that everyone should take a quality daily vitamin supplement.

WHITE CARBOHYDRATES
If it's white, don't bite.

White bread, white pastas and white rice are what you have to avoid. This is a tough one at first, I know. It seems like everything is a white carb. The key is to read the ingredient lists. Look for whole grains and whole wheat products. If it does not say, "whole," it's not. Words to avoid on labels: "bleached", "enriched" and "processed". The more you search, the more you will find that what you have been eating is not what you thought it was. Whole wheat pasta and 100% durum semolina pasta are much easier to find these days. Before you get too uptight, let me gradually phase you into this. The first thing to eliminate is the junk food carbs, like cinnamon rolls or doughnuts. If you want to hold on to your high end pasta with your amazing marinara sauce, I understand. Remember you don't have to do any of this! If pasta is a major deal breaker for you and you really want to enjoy it then that's ok. I would recommend to just cut back like my wife did with cheese. Remember it's a process, so go ahead and enjoy your weekly white pasta splurge and really enjoy it. After time, you may notice it's not that big of a deal, and like my wife, you may decide to give it up all together.

Ben Franklin said it the best: "Eat to live, don't live to eat." These are wise words from a wise man. <u>The cleaner the foods are that you put into your body, the better it runs; it's as simple as that.</u>

REFINED SUGAR
___STOP POISONING YOURSELF!___

You're better off smoking crack cocaine than eating refined sugar. Seriously! Refined sugar is the worst possible thing you can put into your body! It literally kills you. It eats your body from the inside. The scary fact is that in the United States refined sugar is in everything you eat! READ THE LABELS: ketchup, BBQ sauce, breakfast cereals, oatmeal, crackers, salad dressing, etc.! It's disturbing how many foods that boast "honey sweetened" all over the front of the package actually list sugar before honey on the back. Go to the store, grab some "wheat bread" and read how much refined sugar and/or corn syrup is in it! Food manufacturers know that the health-conscious are reading the labels, so they are making it more difficult to identify sugar by giving it fancy names, like "evaporated cane juice/syrup/crystals" and "crystallized cane juice." It also shocks me how much sugar is used in so called "good for you" foods, like yogurt. An average serving of yogurt has between 25 and 45 grams of sugar! There are 4 grams of sugar in a teaspoon, so you do the math! That's like adding 6 to 11 teaspoons of sugar to one cup of yogurt! That's the same amount of sugar as you will find in the average soda pop! JUST READ THE NUTRITION FACTS!

What is great about the human body is that it can heal itself from almost anything. However, if you continue to load it down day after day with poisons and then add stress, not enough sleep, smog, etc., eventually it becomes too much for your body to compensate for and then your systems start to break down, one by one. Specifically, refined sugar destroys your immune system little by little; it's such a gradual process that you don't really notice until it's too late. Help your body help you by eliminating this toxin.

Again, it's all about making a gradual process, slowly start cutting back until finally you start buying sugar-free ketchup, sugar-free BBQ sauce and bread.

So how do you sweeten your foods and drinks? A "sweeter" alternative to refined sugar is Honey or Agave Nectar. Honey tastes fabulous in a variety of foods, but if you are looking for a sweetener that doesn't add any additional taste, you could use the agave; it's just a very sweet, natural low-glycemic index syrup made from the agave plant. You can make some amazing desserts simply by substituting sugar with honey or agave. My Bride no longer puts sugar in her tea; she simply squeezes in some agave and she loves it!

For all you out there like me who were born with a sweet tooth, at the end of this book I will include some of my all-time favorite desserts for you to enjoy. Believe it or not, honey and agave actually taste sweeter than refined sugar, and honey, especially "raw" honey, has some amazing health properties. "Raw" simply refers to a food that has not been heated above 110 degrees, thus preserving the live enzymes that help your body to digest the food. For more information about "raw" foods, see <u>Living on Live Food</u> by Alissa Cohen.

In order to help you make the best food choices, try these tips.

Get rid of the "comfort foods." Sounds easy, but purging the pantry can be a big deal once you have lived a lifetime of bad food habits. It took my wife and me a few years to slowly purge ourselves from junk food, then white carbohydrates and finally sugar. But we did it! (Just don't buy it at the store, and you don't have to worry about not eating it once you get home!) And we are so glad we chose a different way of thinking and eating. Any type of junk food makes me sick now; I don't even want or crave it anymore. If the comfort food isn't in your home, then you won't have anything to "give in" to. When my wife and I first began changing our food choices, sometimes I would just stare at the pantry or even at the open refrigerator and my Bride would ask what I was doing. I was just hoping something "good" would appear. I knew logically it wasn't there, but emotionally I was so used to going to that spot for my "comfort" that my body just went there by instinct. Now we have new comfort foods that are actually beneficial to our bodies and as I said before, you will get some recipes at the end. My favorite dessert now is banana ice cream; once you see the recipe you won't believe what's in it, but when you taste it you will be blown away!

CAN YOU REALLY PREVENT CANCER EATING THIS WAY?

The answer of course is "Yes!" In keeping with our simplicity theme, let's briefly look at how cancer works in your body; the best example is the common cold. When your immune system is low you are more susceptible to catching a cold or any virus. Cancer is the same way; your body is simply unable to fight off the cancer anymore. We all have cancer cells in our body right now, however our bodies are so magnificently designed that we don't even realize we are fighting cancer off every day. Our body naturally regulates and eliminates these damaged and mutated cells so they don't continually grow and divide out of control.

Where everything goes bad is when after years of stress, long term exposure to toxic chemicals like cigarette smoke, exhaust fumes, jet fumes and factory waste compounded with poor food choices with all of its toxic chemicals, our bodies simply say, "Enough." We become so clogged that our bodies can no longer filter out all the toxins and our immune system weakens to a point where it can no longer fight off disease.

It's the same process for the unfortunate and innocent children who contract leukemia and other vicious diseases. Their immune systems were compromised by a genetic flaw or some other reason we are unable to detect. Sadly, in most of these cases, the lives of these precious little ones are too short for our understanding, which is even more motivation for us to make better choices in our lives since we have been blessed with so much.

The best cure for cancer is preventing it in the first place. The best way to prevent it is to focus on things we CAN control. One of the things we have the most control over is what we eat. It all starts with the apple a day.

For some of you, the lack of detailed medical data about cancer in this book may be disturbing. You may also be wondering why I don't cover the different types of cancers like Carcinoma, Sarcoma, Leukemia, Lymphoma or Myeloma.

The answer is simple, the detailed data about cancer fills thousands of medical journals, books, magazines and blogs. People don't need data, the need simple suggestions. Speaking of simple suggestions here is what the Mayo Clinic has on its website, www.mayoclinic.com, for dietary recommendations for cancer survivors word for word:

"Eat 5 or more servings of fruits and vegetables every day, chose healthy fats instead of trans fats, select proteins that are low in saturated fat such as fish, lean meats, eggs, nuts, seeds and legumes, opt for healthy sources of carbohydrates, such as whole grains, legumes, fruits and vegetables. This combination of foods will ensure that you're eating plenty of the vitamins and nutrients you need to help make your body strong."

If the world famous Mayo Clinic is keeping it this simple, shouldn't you?

ACTION STEPS:

#1 Decide not to get overwhelmed and just pick one food to cut back on this week.

#2 Before you eat anything, simply ask yourself, "Do I really want the side effects from this food choice?"

—— ⟋⟍ ——

"For some people, the most exercise they get is jumping to conclusions."

CHAPTER 4

WHAT ABOUT EXERCISE?

As I alluded to at the beginning of this book, no additional exercise is necessary! That's right! Now before you go out and order a new Lazy Boy recliner, let me define "exercise." I define it as something you make yourself do, like going to a gym and getting on a sweat-machine for 30 minutes or taking a class you really don't like. It could be getting on that treadmill or elliptical machine or exercise bike you bought with good intentions, but have grown to hate it as it sits in your bedroom being used as a clothing rack.

So if you agree with my definition, then feel free to burn your gym card or toss your "exercise" contraption. If, however, you do enjoy playing golf or surfing or tennis or basketball or whatever, then by all means do not stop doing it.

Your body burns calories just keeping you alive, and if you have a non-sedentary job or you like playing sports then "exercise", as we have defined it, is not necessary. So what is the next key?

KEY #3:
MOVE!

If you have ever visited a convalescent home, you have heard the term "bed sores." This is a natural reaction when your body sits too long. I'm not talking about "exercising," but moving is the key. As I said before, your body burns calories just keeping your heart pumping and any extra movement you can do will be <u>extremely beneficial</u>. An example of "moving": Walking. I would not consider taking a walk around the block "exercise," but it keeps your body moving. Our lifestyle has become so sedentary for most people that we have to offset that with conscious movement. Think about it: we drive to work and look for the closest parking spot, then we sit on our "assets" all day in the cubicle, then we drive home and sit in front of the T.V.

I read an article about a company that has all their meetings while walking instead of sitting. They even have treadmills for desks instead of traditional desks. They only go 1 mph, but they keep moving. Now should you go take your treadmill from your house and stick it in your cubicle? Sure!

Here are some other "moving" suggestions:

Take the stairs! Simply take the stairs every chance you get and you will be surprised at how much stronger this will make you. If you work in an office building, take the stairs every day: when you arrive, when you go in between the floors for breaks, lunch, etc. The first week or two may be tough, but soon enough you will see how much stronger you become.

Walk to work, or ride a bike if possible.

Walk at lunch. You don't need to walk a marathon, just a few blocks every day.

When you get home walk around the block <u>before</u> you sit down to watch T.V.

At work move your printer to a location away from your desk. Force yourself to get out of your chair each time you print something. If this is not workable, simply get up and stretch every hour. You don't need to do a yoga routine, just a simple reach your hands to the sky and get on your tip-toes is all you need.

When you get home, walk around the block <u>before</u> you sit down to watch T.V. This is not a typo; I am just making sure you got the message.

Get up at each commercial break. Simply get off your assets during each commercial and do a simple stretch. I could give you 10,000 ideas; the key is to just remember to move your body; that's what it was made to do.

As I said before; you don't have to do any of this. If you just eat fruit everyday from the time you wake up until noon you will look and feel 10,000 times better. However, if you add in the suggestions of this chapter about moving your body, you will see your results compound.

ACTION STEPS:

#1 Take the stairs instead of the elevator or escalator.

#2 Stand up and stretch at each commercial break when you watch T.V.

"There's more to life than being really, really, really good looking."
– Zoolander

CHAPTER 5

GENETICS AND HOW TO WORK WITH THEM

In the beginning of this book I shared with you my ignorance in my early bodybuilding career about genetics. I truly believed a horse jockey, for example, could be an NFL Linemen if he simply lifted enough weights. The reverse of this thinking is also just as ignorant. How many times have you heard the overweight guy or gal say, "I'm just big boned"? The truth of the matter is being overweight or underweight has everything to do with your eating habits and emotional stability (more on emotional stability in Key# 5), but this leads us into:

KEY #4:
KNOW YOUR BODY TYPE.

The three main body types are Ectomorph, Mesomorph and Endomorph. Relax, I will explain what the prefixes mean: ecto- means small, meso- is medium and endo- is large. Now let me first address the ladies.

Let me explain it to you, ladies. Look at your wrist; if you have big, stocky grandparents or parents, typically you have much bigger wrists than your petite 5'1" and 99 pound friend. A great example is the T.V. show "The View". Elisabeth Hasselbeck, who we had the pleasure of befriending before she was selected to be on the show, is a very petite, or Ectomorph, woman. However, Joy Behar is about the same height, but much stockier.

Another great example from the same show is Star Jones, and her amazing transformation! She could have used the "big boned" excuse, but now that she lost 150 pounds, look at how small she is! She made a choice and lost the weight.

Lastly, ladies, take a look at Serena Williams, the professional tennis player; she is in world class shape! But her body structure is not super lean and skinny. Look at her sister, Venus: her body type is much leaner and less stocky. Both women are in fabulous shape, but their body structures are very different.

OK, Guys! Now it's your turn. Look at a typical NFL cornerback or wide-receiver, then look at a NFL offensive lineman, they are clearly different body structures. If you ever get a close up look at an of-fensive lineman's wrists, they are huge! They are Endomorphs. It's literally in their genes.

You can look healthy and in shape no matter what your body structure. Take some well known Endomorphs for example, bodybuilders Arnold Schwarzenegger or Lou Ferrigno. Lou is 6'5 and 300 pounds with only 5% body-fat. These guys have proven "big boned" does not mean "fat." Whatever your body type is, you CAN look great!

The key is to understand what your body is capable of and not get depressed if you're not able to fit in a size 2, ladies. Guys, the same with you, if your body structure is like Shaquille O'Neal, then you are not going to be able to get a body like Kobe Bryant. However, if you look at pictures of Shaq when he was "really in shape," he looked great for what he had to work with. Just be the best you and the "One Day Diet" will make it easier.

ACTION STEPS:

#1 Identify your body type.

#2 Do the best you can with the body that God gave you.

"It's not what you're eating, it's what's eating you."
– Janet Greeson Ph.D.

CHAPTER 6

WHAT'S EATING YOU?

You may have heard the saying, "It's not what you're eating, it's what's eating you." I agree to an extent. We all know that what you put in your body determines what your body looks like and how you feel. However, there is more to it than just food. This leads to:

KEY #5:
EVERYTHING IS CONNECTED

Now, this could be an entire book on its own, so I'm just going to touch on a few ideas. The reason I'm even opening this "can of worms" is because I have seen people that had amazing looking bodies, who ate well and were in great shape, but then all of a sudden they turned to mush. An example of this is Oprah; sometimes she is in amazing shape and other times she plumps up, why?

I have a few answers for you that I will briefly cover.

SELF IMAGE:

People subconsciously always revert to what <u>they believe</u> is true. It doesn't matter what the real truth is; it matters what they believe. So if people don't love themselves and they think they are worthless, they will end up being 40 or even 400 pounds overweight.

Lottery winners are a perfect example of this. In their minds they are just average people making $30,000 a year. Suddenly, they get $30 million and they simply self destruct, go bankrupt and in a matter of a few years they are right back to making $30,000 a year again.

Your self-image is like a thermostat, so if you if you set it at 70 degrees and it drops down to 64 or 65 degrees, the heater kicks on. For example, 99.9%

of you reading this book are not homeless. Why? Well, when things get a little cold your thermostat kicks on and you do what it takes to pay your rent or mortgage or move to a smaller place. Whatever you need to do you do it because your self-image is that of someone living in a house or an apartment, not on the street.

Another great example is people who are suffering from bulimia. They are simply skin and bones and yet they think, feel and see themselves as FAT. The truth is irrelevant to them; it's all about how they perceive themselves or their self-image.

STRESS:

Your body releases cortisol when you are stressed, to help your system cope with the situations. The two main side effects of an excess of cortisol are that it eats muscle and it causes the body to store fat, mostly around the mid section; the more stressed you are, the more fat it stores. This can be the result of emotional stress. Just look at the typical 30 to 40 year old executive. He has a wife, kids, mortgage, stressful job, and what do you see but the rapidly growing belly. It can also be caused by physical stress. Look at the hard core marathoners, they all have this belly fat and, other than their legs, hardly any muscle tone.

UNFORGIVENESS:

As the best selling author of <u>Take Action Now-How to Live Your Dream in Less Than 3 Weeks</u>, (available on Amazon & Kindle), I dedicate a whole chapter to this subject. I joke that most people are carrying around 40 pounds of unforgiveness. Everything affects everything else. Women know this, but guys are such "masters at compartmentalizing" that they often fool themselves. However, your body will not be fooled and it will pay a huge price. Carrying around anger, resentment and hurt towards another person, or persons, WILL TAKE ITS TOLL. It starts as a simple lowering of your immune system and then it can spread to be chronic pain or even cancer. There are countless stories of miracle healings after people have finally forgiven others. I'm a huge believer in God's miracles, but if you really look at it, forgiveness itself could be a miracle of its own.

If this has struck a chord with you I highly recommend my book (Take Action Now), as I cover specific action steps and more details on how to let go and forgive.

ACTION STEPS:

#1 Forgive someone!

#2 If we all practiced the "eye for an eye" principal everyone would be blind.

FINAL THOUGHTS...

As the #1 Online Life Coach (www.lifecoach5.com), I'm often asked for some free advice from friends and family, etc. and I'm honored to help wherever I can. One day my dental hygienist was cleaning my teeth and asked me some Life Coaching questions about her health. Since I was in the dental chair being worked on I had to choose my words carefully. She was talking about how people make excuses about brushing and flossing, such as "I don't have time," etc., until finally after experiencing some heavy drilling and a few root canals, they get with the program. What was interesting was that in her mind, since she is a dental hygienist, there is no excuse for not brushing and flossing. After a few mumbled words and questions from me, it then dawned on her that if she thought that same way about the foods she was eating, (that there is no excuse for not making good food choices), she would be at the health and weight goals she really wanted.

That's what great Life Coaching does; it allows you to own the solution and break out of your limited thinking.

If you are excited about getting World Class Life Coaching, but the initial investment is something that is holding you back, join the thousands of others who take advantage of our online Life Coaching at www.lifecoach5.com. As a personal gift to you, we would like to extend a 30 day free trial offer. Simply e-mail <u>coach@lifecoach5.</u> <u>com</u> and put "One Day Diet FREE 30 day" in the subject.

If you would like to see if you qualify for our personal Life Coaching programs, please call 1-877-WOW- EVAN or 310-750-6219.

E-mail: coach@lifecoach5.com

As promised here are a few of my favorite recipes...

Banana Ice Cream

2-3 very ripe bananas, peeled, chopped in 1 inch sections and frozen (Tip: I usually will freeze <u>8-10</u> bananas at a time, place in zipper freezer bag, and lay it <u>flat</u> in the freezer, or else it will freeze in big clumps that are hard to break up.)

Put frozen banana chunks in a food processor or a hard core blender. Please note cheapo blenders cannot handle this and will die an ugly death. Then blend, blend, blend until creamy. (For the first minute or so, it will just look kind of chunky, but if you are patient and keep pushing it into the blade with the tamper, it will suddenly "cream up," you then have perfectly textured and creamy "ice cream".) Most of you reading this will not believe it until you see it and when you finally taste it, you will be blown away! For a little variety, you may add: blueberries, cocoa powder, vanilla, honey, cinnamon, etc.

<u>Fruit Cobbler</u>

Preheat oven to 350 degrees.

2 – 10 oz. bags frozen fruit, thawed, or you can use fresh (blueberries, blackberries, cherries, peaches, or mix two different ones together)

½ cup agave nectar

2 tbsp. flour

Mix thoroughly in bowl and pour into oiled 9x9 glass baking dish; set aside.

1 cup rolled uncooked oats

½ cup flour

½ cup nugget cereal (like Grape Nuts or Kashi)

¼ tsp. salt

Mix these dry ingredients, and then add:

2-3 tbsp. canola oil

2 tbsp. agave nectar

Spread evenly over top of fruit mixture. Bake until slightly golden, 25-30 minutes. Let cool slightly and enjoy warm.

Applesauce Cake/Cupcakes

Preheat oven to 350 degrees.

Mix dry ingredients in medium bowl, and set aside.

2 cups flour

½ tsp. cinnamon

¼ tsp. nutmeg

¼ tsp. salt

1 ½ tsp. baking powder

½ tsp. baking soda

Mix wet ingredients together in a large bowl.

½ cup canola oil

2/3 cup honey

1 egg

¾ -1 cup applesauce

¼ tsp. almond extract

Slowly add dry mixture to wet mixture and blend, but do not over stir.

Pour into oiled baking pan/cupcake pan and bake 25-30 minutes for cake, 20-25 minutes for cupcakes. You know when it is truly ready if you pierce with knife and it comes out clean. Cool and enjoy!

ACTION STEPS GUIDE SHEET:

Chapter 1

#1 Find a picture in a magazine of what you want your body to look like. Cut it out and post it somewhere you will see it every day.

#2 Start with the apple a day theory. Just decide you will eat one apple sometime today. Then manage that decision tomorrow and choose to eat an apple. You may want to go to the store and buy 7 or 8 apples so you can have them available.

Chapter 2

#1 Stock up on fruit today so you will have enough to follow through with eating fruit only until noon every day.

#2 Plan ahead on taking fruits with you that are not as messy as others for when you go to work, or wherever you travel before noon every day. Eat the messy ones at home.

Chapter 3

#1 Decide not to get overwhelmed and just choose one food to cut back on this week.

#2 Before you eat anything, simply ask yourself, "Do I really want the side effects from this food choice?"

Chapter 4

#1 Take the stairs instead of the elevator or escalator.

#2 Stand up and stretch at each commercial break when you watch T.V.

Chapter 5

#1 Identify your body type.

#2 Do the best you can with the body that God gave you.

Chapter 6

#1 Forgive someone!

#2 If we all practiced the "eye for an eye" principal everyone would be blind.

www.theonedaydiet.com

To contact Evan for speaking engagements call:
1-877-WOW-EVAN
or e-mail:
evan@evanmoney.com
www.evanmoney.com

THE ONE DAY DIET

How to Live a Cancer Prevention Lifestyle

EVAN MONEY

"Evan Money is one of those rare individuals who puts his beliefs into action; he will teach you to do the same. Evan walks the walk and that is what makes him so special. He has my highest recommendation!"

Dr. Keith Phillips - President, World Impact

"Evan's personality contagiously inspires everyone who comes in contact with him. His focused and dedicated approach motivates and encourages others to maximize their own individual abilities and realize positive growth in their lives, and leads them to be the best at what they do."

Jeff Harlow - Arena Football Team Owner / Boxing Promoter

"I have known Evan and his family for years. Honest, Creative, Dynamic, Expressive, when Evan speaks you want to listen. He thinks big, dreams big and then he moves and makes his dreams a reality. Adding action to ideas? - Evan lives it. If you can catch just a little of his fire, a little of his passion, it could make life oh so much more interesting."

Dr. Douglas Holtzinger - *Founder, Back Care Institute*

"Experts and Educators thrive on making simple things complicated, Communicators make complicated things simple."
– Dr. John C. Maxwell

—— ❧❧ ——

"I didn't know I had a headache until the pain stopped."

"Eat to live, don't live to eat."
– Benjamin Franklin

---

*"For some people, the
most exercise they get is
jumping to conclusions."*

———— ⁊⁊ ————

*"There's more to life
than being really, really,
really good looking."
– Zoolander*

———— ⚬⚬ ————

*"It's not what you're eating,
it's what's eating you."
– Janet Greeson Ph.D.*

NOTES

www.theonedaydiet.com

NOTES

NOTES

www.theonedaydiet.com

NOTES

www.theonedaydiet.com